Joseane de Araújo Benvenuto
Nely Cristina M. Caires

Level of satisfaction of Total Prosthesis users: UNIP- Manaus

Joseane de Araújo Benvenuto
Nely Cristina M. Caires

Level of satisfaction of Total Prosthesis users: UNIP-Manaus

Self-assessment using the OHIP-14

Imprint

Any brand names and product names mentioned in this book are subject to trademark, brand or patent protection and are trademarks or registered trademarks of their respective holders. The use of brand names, product names, common names, trade names, product descriptions etc. even without a particular marking in this work is in no way to be construed to mean that such names may be regarded as unrestricted in respect of trademark and brand protection legislation and could thus be used by anyone.

Cover image: www.ingimage.com

This book is a translation from the original published under ISBN 978-613-9-66233-3.

Publisher:
Sciencia Scripts
is a trademark of
Dodo Books Indian Ocean Ltd. and OmniScriptum S.R.L publishing group

120 High Road, East Finchley, London, N2 9ED, United Kingdom
Str. Armeneasca 28/1, office 1, Chisinau MD-2012, Republic of Moldova, Europe
Printed at: see last page
ISBN: 978-620-7-99466-3

ABSTRACT: The aim of this study was to assess the self-perception of complete denture wearers who sought care at the Universidade Paulista (UNIP) - Manaus campus in order to have a new denture made. The project was approved by the CEP of UNIP. Twelve patients took part in the study and the OH IP-14 questionnaire was used to assess and measure the level of satisfaction of the patients in question after six months of using the new prosthesis. After the stipulated time, a new interview was carried out using the same questionnaire for comparison, using the Wilcoxon and MacNemar tests as statistical tools. In general, around 91.6% (11) were satisfied and reported a slight discomfort with chewing, due to the regional diet, which consists mainly of manioc flour and fish. And 8.3% (1) of the patients reported being dissatisfied after delivery, but did not return for the necessary adjustments and returned for the final interview. The conclusion is that it is important to restore the patient's aesthetics and masticatory function, as these are important factors for quality of life, and that there was also a change in self-esteem when patients showed satisfaction with the result of their new dental prosthesis.

Keywords: Quality of Life, Total Prosthesis, Patient Satisfaction.

SUMMARY

CHAPTER 1

INTRODUCTION

For many years, dental treatment, even before the implementation of the Unified Health System (SUS), was in most cases mutilating, even if the correct procedure was conservative (SILVA, 2010). This was due to the high demand from young and adult patients seeking the public service, with caries and periodontal disease being described as the main causes of tooth loss. This fact is now quantified by the number of edentulous people in the country (FRAZÃO, 2003).

In Brazil, in particular, the total loss of teeth (edentulism) is still accepted by society as something normal and common as a person gets older, and not as a reflection of the lack of preventive public health policies, aimed mainly at adults, so that they can keep their teeth until they are older. Epidemiological surveys show that there is no restorative treatment available to the majority of the population. Public services carry out mass extractions and provide the elderly population with only emergency care, causing the need for rehabilitative treatment to accumulate and reach high levels. With the high levels of extractions carried out, there is a high demand for prosthetic treatments, which are not offered to the population (COLUSSI, 2014).

In the long term, tooth loss affects the individual's life, causing damage to chewing, phonetics and aesthetics (ETTINGER, 1997). Mastication is the first step towards digestion, and for this to take place, teeth are needed, so that grinding takes place and food is swallowed and digested in the future. Often, edentulous patients change their diet, making adaptations due to masticatory impairment, opting for softer food that is easier to chew (SIQUEIRA, 2010). Speech is another constant problem, as some sounds are lost, and aesthetics, which is important in daily social interaction, affects the self-esteem of the edentulous (PESQUEIRO, 2005).

In dentistry there are several options for rehabilitation and one of them is the mucosupported removable complete denture, which can artificially restore tooth loss (PESQUEIRO 2005). It is relatively inexpensive and the moulding and fabrication technique is simple when compared to other forms of rehabilitation and can be carried out by a general dentist.

The rehabilitation of patients who need prostheses is of the utmost importance, as they are given back their stomatognathic function, which brings with it significant improvements in their personal and social lives. The search for a better life expectancy has been increasing over the years and has helped in the search for rehabilitation (SIQUEIRA 2010).

Various factors influence the level of satisfaction of rehabilitated patients. These factors are related to retention, stability, adaptation and occlusion, since the masticatory function is considered to be the most important for denture wearers. It can be said that rehabilitating an edentulous patient will restore facial harmony and physical and emotional well-being (LUCENA, 2010).

Despite the legal guarantees, the growth in resources and the expansion of services, the implementation of public policies that include the elderly in oral health actions is still incipient in order to ensure active public-governmental commitment to the elderly and their health and thus transform the epidemiological reality. The Brazilian state, despite proclaiming the universality and comprehensiveness of health actions and positive signals from the public administration, continues to exclude the vast majority of the elderly from oral health care. In order to change this reality, it is necessary to develop a critical sense, research and promote the adoption of new practices, build differentiated strategies, promote community involvement, integrate actions and mobilise resources, always with a view to ageing healthily (MELLO, 2008).

In view of the above, this study aims to assess the level of satisfaction of patients rehabilitated in the Total Prosthesis clinic of the UNIP Dentistry Clinic Manaus campus in 2011, and to measure the dimensions of the group's quality of life, using the OHIP-14 scores. The study was carried out in two stages: the first interview took place in October 2011 and the follow-up took place between May and July 2012, six months after delivery.

The study was completed in 2013 and re-edited in 2018 to produce this book. The studies cited for scientific knowledge on the subject were selected according to the year of the first edition.

CHAPTER 2

DEVELOPMENT

2.1 Elderly Health - Main Clinical Manifestations

Ageing is a natural process of life, but it is necessary to know the most appropriate way to age healthily and with a quality of life that is favourable to the age of the elderly person according to their needs and limitations. Dawilibi et al (2013) define "ageing as a multifaceted socio-vital process throughout the life course". Old age denotes the state of "being old", a condition that results from the ageing process that generations have experienced and are experiencing within diverse social, political and individual contexts. There is a difficulty in defining quality of life, as it is a subjective construct and determined by numerous interconnected variables throughout life, including human ageing. Understanding ageing as an irreversible phenomenon is of the utmost importance so that everyone - health professionals, the government, society in general and the elderly themselves - sees old age not as finitude, but as a moment in the life cycle that requires specific care, which can and should be enjoyed with quality.

The study by Dawalibi et al (2013) analysed 69 articles on ageing and quality of life. The authors begin their text by revealing that by 2025 the number of elderly people is expected to exceed 30 million, and old age may be accompanied by high levels of chronic diseases as well as health and well-being. It is important to improve the socio-economic conditions of emerging countries, such as Brazil, in order to provide quality of life for the elderly. elderly in their old age. In Brazil, the increase in the elderly population has been happening rapidly and progressively, without any corresponding change in living conditions. In which they cite the World Health Organisation's (WHO, 2005) proposal as a real example of the recommendations, emphasising that ageing well is not just the responsibility of the individual, but a process that must be supported by public policies and social and health initiatives throughout the course of life. In order to age healthily, it is essential to increase the opportunities for individuals to opt for a more appropriate lifestyle, including changes in eating habits and regular physical activity, and consequently control of physical and psychological health.

Brito et. al (2013), when carrying out a bibliographical survey on population ageing and the challenges for public health, revealed that the Brazilian epidemiological situation has a triple burden of disease, as it involves, at the same time: an unfinished agenda of infections, malnutrition and reproductive health problems; a strong growth in external causes; and the challenge of chronic diseases and their risk factors, such as smoking, overweight, obesity, physical inactivity, stress and inadequate nutrition. Successful ageing therefore requires not only public health policies, but also the health sector to be prepared to respond in the fields of prevention and health promotion for older people. Programmes aimed at the elderly must meet their specific needs in terms of physiological, psychological and social aspects, as well as understanding their profile and social reality. The analyses of the articles led to the following conclusions: the high cost of elderly health care for health services; the importance of interdisciplinary action in caring for the elderly; and new models of care that have been applied to overcome these challenges.

Mello et al (2008), mentioning the new Brazilian demographic profile associated with an ageing population, has led to changes in morbidity, disability and mortality patterns. In addition to the occurrence of infectious diseases, the prevalence of chronic non-communicable diseases is increasing and, therefore, the importance of the respective risk factors, which require preventive action. The changing pattern is no different in oral health, where the epidemiological profile of oral health in the Brazilian population is also undergoing changes, especially in the levels of dental caries, the most prevalent oral disease. Between 1986 and 1996, there was a sharp decrease of approximately 50% in the respective years, although the gain was uneven, confirming the social determination of the health-disease process. At older ages, there is an increase in root caries, periodontal diseases, oral mucosa pathologies and the need for prostheses. They also point out that the absence of state coverage is partially covered by a private system of provision and production of dental services, competing for and serving the segment of demand that is able to pay, leaving a huge population excluded from meeting their most basic oral health care needs. Thus, access to and the benefits provided by new technologies are restricted to elderly people who can afford private market services, or those who have the support of a corporate health plan, which is generally rare for those who have reached the elderly stage.

Shinkai (2000), in his bibliographical study on the role of dentistry in comprehensive health care for the elderly, states that there are few epidemiological studies on the oral health conditions of the elderly, making it impossible to establish priorities and develop coherent care actions. Even in developed countries, geriatric dentistry was only consolidated in the 1970s and the following decade. The same author cites as examples the events related to the founding of the International Association of Gerontology (IAG) in 1983; the first meeting of the International Dental Federation's working group on the oral health of the elderly in 1988; and the development of programmes and curricular modules in geriatric dentistry for dental schools in the United States in the 80s. In Brazil, Albuquerque suggested the inclusion of geriatric dentistry in the dental curriculum in 1982. In addition to the formal inclusion of geriatrics and gerontology in dental school curricula, Shinkai believes that there is also an urgent need for human resources training in geriatric dentistry for the entire oral health team, not just dental surgeons, in order to make it possible to provide care for the elderly population on a large scale.

Given the natural process of ageing, individual biological processes occur naturally and are accompanied by social and demographic changes. Over the years, vocal deterioration is typical and has a major impact, reinforcing the stereotype of the elderly. Based on this vocal deterioration, Menezes (2007) carried out a cross-sectional clinical study with anamnesis and phonoaudiological assessment on a random sample of 48 elderly individuals living in the Francisco Azevedo Elderly House in Belo Horizonte. It assessed the perceptual-auditory form of the vocal characteristics of institutionalised elderly people, identified the properties that interfere with communication and correlated them with the assessment of the structures of the stomagnatic system and the speech pattern. Among the participants, 85 per cent of the elderly had no natural teeth and 60 per cent wear dentures. The results of the perceptual-auditory assessment of vocal quality showed a predominance of hoarse vocal quality (70.8%), moderate vocal quality (33.3%), reduced loudness (56.2%), low pitch (62.5%) and reduced maximum times (81.2%). This study can verify isolated data that may be due to tooth loss, which can alter muscle function, reducing facial muscle tone. These alterations are: a higher prevalence of altered tongue posture, characterised mainly by anteriorisation and resting on the floor of the mouth; and altered tongue mobility, such as tongue tip elevation and lowering, lateralisation, palate sweep and rotation. The conclusion is that this population needs interdisciplinary work with speech therapists, dentists, doctors, nutritionists and psychologists.

Shinkai (2000) mentions that from an anatomical and functional point of view, dentistry's specific area of activity is the stomatognathic system, comprising teeth, periodontal tissues, oral mucosa, tongue, salivary glands, maxilla and mandible, masticatory muscles and the temporomandibular joint (TMJ). With ageing, anatomical changes are common, but these do not necessarily constitute an imbalance in the health-disease process. When it comes to the oral problems of the elderly, which are actually complications of pathological processes due to poor oral hygiene, iatrogenesis, lack of guidance and interest in oral health, they are generally associated with non-access to dental services. With ageing, there is also a predisposition to some morbidities, such as oral cancer, which has age as a risk factor. He also reports on the most prevalent oral problems in the elderly: coronal and root caries, periodontopathies, edentulism, dental wear (attrition, abrasions and erosions), soft tissue lesions (ulcerations, traumatic and drug-induced inflammatory hyperplasia, infections, etc.), xerostomia, orofacial pain, temporomandibular disorders (TMD), occlusion problems and oral cancer (not listed in order of prevalence or clinical relevance).

Bomfim (2008), in order to identify the prevalence of mucosal lesions in the oral cavity of denture wearers and their relationship with hygiene habits, examined 94 individuals of both genders with dentures who were treated at the Prosthetic Clinic/DOR/UFPB and at the Prosthetic Services of Cruz das Armas, João Pessoa/PB. After collecting the data by means of a semiological clinical examination by a single examiner, the gender, type of prosthesis, form of hygiene, frequency of time wearing the prosthesis, type of lesion and description of the lesion were recorded on a clinical form. The results were that 41.5% of the patients were male and 58.5% female; of those with clinically visible lesions, 69.1% were male, 16.9%

female and 83.1% female. The general aspects related to dissatisfaction with the prostheses assessed were 54.2% broken; 71.2% stained; 73.4% visible biofilm; 59.5% tooth wear; 73.4% lack of stability and 47.8% had occlusion problems. When it came to occlusion problems, the data was 25.5% referring to top-to-bottom occlusion; 15.9% mandibular protrusion; occlusion only in the anterior region; 9.5% open bite; 3.18% occlusion only on one side of the prosthesis. The prevalence of mucosal lesions was 69.1%, the most frequent being prosthetic stomatitis (PS) with 44.6% of the cases presented. Of these, 61.7% of patients slept with their dentures in; 53.1% had visible biofilm on their dentures; 67% of cases were female and in all cases the lesion was located on the palate. The second most frequent lesion seen was Inflammatory Fibrous Hyperplasia (IFH), present in 42.5% of patients, where 39.3% had a lack of stability in the prosthesis, 46.8% were female and 45.7% of cases occurred on the upper alveolar ridge. Other lesions diagnosed included: Flaccid ridge (16%); Angular cheilitis (12.7%); Compression area (7.4%); Traumatic ulcer (2.1%); Fibroma (2.1%); Lichen planus (3.2%); and Geographic tongue (2.1%). No neoplasms were found in this study.

In the book Saúde do Idoso (Health of the Elderly), Chaimowicz et. al (2013), Ribeiro, the author of a chapter in the book, tells the story of a fictional lady called Dona Josefina, with an average age of 80, who was found by a team of health professionals in very poor health. Amongst many other health complications, she says that she had difficulty chewing food, thus changing her diet and jeopardising her nutrition. Like Mrs Josefina, many elderly people suffer from major health problems, especially oral health. These include preventive maintenance of prostheses - partial dentures and full dentures; complications from insufficient prevention; and oral cancer. When referring to the preventive maintenance of dentures, especially partial dentures, she mentions the importance of caring for the abutment teeth, as without proper maintenance these teeth can develop carious lesions. It also highlights the greater frequency of risk factors for caries and periodontal disease that can affect the elderly, such as hyposalivation, reduced manual dexterity, cognitive problems and dietary changes caused by tooth loss. Full dentures require corrective maintenance because the alveolar ridge undergoes a continuous process of formation and resorption. When ill-fitting, they compromise the aesthetics and mastication of the elderly. There is a bidirectional relationship between the masticatory capacity, diet and nutritional condition of the elderly. Because of these complications, the elderly suffer from weight loss due to nutritional problems that can interfere with the adaptation of the prosthesis; on the other hand, when the prosthesis is poorly adapted, it can lead to nutritional problems. When it comes to complications that are insufficiently preventable, mucosal alterations, due to their impact on quality of life and nutritional conditions, poorly adapted prostheses or poor hygiene conditions. The main mucosal alterations are: inflammatory hyperplasia and pressure ulcers, which are related to poor adaptation and maintenance of prostheses, as well as candidiasis, which is related to poor hygiene. Finally, oral cancer, which is highly prevalent in soft tissues, emphasises the need for regular oral examinations to prevent it. It is strategically important to screen for oral neoplasms, especially in elderly people with neuropsychiatric disorders (depression and dementia) or vision and manual dexterity disorders.

2.1 - Edentulism in Brazil

Edentulism is the total absence of teeth, which damages health, function, aesthetics and psychological health. In an interview with www.portaldoenvelhecimento.org.br Dr Fernando Luiz Brunette Montenegro said that the reason why so many elderly people are edentulous is not because there is no technique or material for non-radical treatment, but because it is "easy, quick and cheap". He added that it wasn't dentistry that had changed, but the possibility of access.

Shinkai, 2000, carried out a bibliographical study and states that all his studies show a high prevalence of edentulism, dental caries and periodontopathies, reflecting the failure or non-existence of dental care for the population analysed. He emphasises that in Brazil, interest in the oral health of the elderly only began in the 70s.

Brazil has seen an increase in life expectancy. Data released by the Brazilian Institute of Geography and Statistics (IBGE) showed that in 1950 this expectation was 43.3 years and in 2012 it was 74 years and 29 days, which shows us the need for health policies aimed at this age group, and therefore for the rehabilitation of edentulous patients.

An epidemiological study carried out in 2010 by the Ministry of Health through the

Smiling Brazil programme, in which the 26 state capitals plus the Federal District took part. It found that among the elderly aged between 65 and 74, more than three million need full dentures in both arches and around four million need partial dentures in one of the arches (SB-BRASIL, 2010).

Comparing 2003, the year in which the same epidemiological study was also carried out, with 2010, around 24% versus 23% wore dentures on one arch in their respective years, as well as 16% versus 15% wore full dentures on both arches. In the same study, adults aged 35 and 44 had increased access to caries treatment and fewer teeth were being extracted because of the disease (SB-BRASIL 2010).

According to Pinto (2000), edentulous elderly patients are no longer interested in oral health programmes, however, given the influence of oral health on general health, this group represents a priority for dentistry. Tertiary prevention via maintenance of prosthetic appliances is essential among some of the health promotion measures for the elderly. As well as programmes aimed at maintaining natural teeth, reducing edentulism rates.

The damage caused by oral diseases increases with age, increasing the use of prostheses, and these services are generally not offered by the public health system. In the case of edentulism (absence of teeth), the use of dental services is important to assess the need for prostheses, as well as their replacement in order to diagnose pathologies such as oral cancer at an early stage. A comparative study between toothed and toothless elderly people, carried out in 2002/2003 by the Ministry of Health, called SB Brasil, was reported by Martins et. al (2007), in which participants in the oral health survey in the south-eastern region of Brazil were restricted to having used the services for less than a year and were compared to those who had used them for more than a year. A total of 1,014 elderly people aged between 65 and 74 took part in the study. Of these, 345 were dentate - with at least one tooth in the oral cavity - and 669 were edentulous - with no teeth at all; respectively, the prevalence of use was 32 per cent and 11 per cent. Of the dentate patients, 111 (32%) had used the services for less than a year and 76 (11%) had used the services in the same period. The study's analysis shows that the proportion of elderly people who had used dental services for less than a year was very low and that the factors associated with use between dentate and edentate people show differences related to inequity in the use of dental services. Among the factors of inequality was the presence of individual factors, including the availability of resources to explain dental services. Although it is essential to guarantee the group's access to dental services, especially among those with edentulous teeth, there was a tendency to use services only when the oral health situation is critical, with the presence of pain, appearance perceived as very bad or bad, or when they have oral problems.

Silva et al (2010) carried out a study in Belo Horizonte, at the Faculty of Dentistry of the Federal University of Minas Gerais, to assess the impact of tooth loss on quality of life. They selected fifty patients, users of the Public Health Service, undergoing treatment for the insertion or replacement of a pair of dentures. During the interview, the Oral Health Impact Profile (OHIP-14) was applied and sociodemographic data was collected. The results were as follows: the sample was made up of 82% females and 18% males; the average age of the participants was 59.1 years; the sociodemographic characteristics revealed that only 24% of the sample were working and the rest were not working or were retired; the dimensions with the greatest impact on the quality of life of the interviewees were observed in psychological discomfort, pain and psychological inability; the total loss of teeth did not represent an obstacle to their social interaction; for both the ten patients who achieved the highest OHIP-14 scores and the ten participants who achieved the lowest scores, the questions with the highest scores referred to discomfort when eating food because of problems with their mouth or dentures - the pain dimension - and feelings of shame caused by their mouth or dentures - the psychological inability dimension. Of those interviewed, 80% reported that they had never faced any problems in relation to the disability dimensions; the questions referred to the perception that life was made worse because of the problems caused by their teeth, mouth or dentures; 79% of people had already been irritated by other people because of problems with their teeth, mouth or dentures and had found it difficult to carry out their daily activities because of problems with their teeth, mouth or dentures. Regarding the functional limitation dimension, 63 per cent of the interviewees reported difficulty in speaking some words because of problems with their teeth, mouth or dentures. They concluded that in the group studied, the absence of teeth or the use of inadequate prostheses has little effect on their ability to carry out their daily activities and to interact in their environment, although it does have a negative impact on some dimensions of quality of life, which were psychological discomfort, pain and psychological inability. This information is important for adequately training the professionals responsible for caring for patients who have experienced or are about to experience total or partial tooth loss.

Medeiros (2012) points out that the total loss of teeth is still seen as a natural process of ageing, and not as a consequence of diseases such as caries and periodontal disease associated with the lack of preventive programmes and policies designed for the adult and elderly population. Social inequalities interfere not only with oral health, but also with the general health of populations, so that individuals living in areas with large differences in income have worse oral conditions compared to those with a similar socioeconomic situation, but who live in regions with less economic disparity. The World Health Organisation (WHO) states that for a country to change its health situation, it must take action to reduce social inequalities. Specifically in oral health, socioeconomic inequality is a risk factor for most oral diseases and for indicators of access to and use of dental services, both at an ecological and individual level.

Martins et al (2008) state that edentulism is a characteristic of the Brazilian population and is prevalent and irreversible among those affected. It is important to know the factors associated with the use of dental services in this specific population, in order to contribute to oral health policies that can improve quality of life.

2.2 . Total Prosthesis: Brazil and the North and Northeast Regions

According to Turano and Turano (2002), prosthesis "is the replacement of lost or unformed tissue". The word derives from the Greek: por diante, in place of; and *thesis, to* place. Etymologically, putting something in place of something else". He also mentions that in 1692, Antón Nuck built the first known lower denture from a piece of hippopotamus molar.

In Belo Horizonte, Maruch et. al (2009) carried out an epidemiological study of elderly people who took part in the Belo Horizonte City Council's Coexistence Group in 2004 and needed rehabilitation. They used the Geriatric Assessment Index (GOHAI), made up of twelve questions divided into three domains (physical, psychosocial and pain) and the results obtained were: 26% reported "always" having limitations in masticatory function; 19% said they "sometimes" had difficulty swallowing; 69% "never" restricted their social contacts because of their appearance, and 22% "never" restricted their social contacts because of their appearance.

"always" used medication to relieve pain or discomfort. When the removable total dental prostheses (TP) were examined, it was found that they had limitations which had an impact on quality of life, thus indicating the need to invest in health promotion programmes to preserve natural dental elements.

In João Pessoa, Paraíba, Furtado et al (2000) used the Geriatric Oral Health Assessment Index (GOHAI) to examine 24 elderly people, with a mean age of 73.4 years and the majority female. They reported that the use of prostheses (complete and partial dentures) was more frequent in the upper arch, with complete dentures being more common than partial dentures in both arches. When asked about limitations in the type and quality of food they ate due to problems with their teeth and dentures, most of the elderly (66.7%) had never experienced this type of limitation. For the majority of the elderly people examined (87.5%), their oral condition did not pose any problems for their social life, nor did it interfere with their self-esteem (66.7%). The majority (66.7%) felt no pain or discomfort in their teeth or dentures. Overall, 54% of the elderly had a low self-perception of oral health.

Using the same GOHAI questionnaire, Silva et al (2006) carried out a study to see if there was a relationship between self-perceived oral health and overall satisfaction with life, with 17 women over the age of 60 who came to the Total Prosthesis Clinic at the Piracicaba School of Dentistry (SP). The results showed that the average age of the patients was 67.88 years and that 58.9% of these women rated their oral health as low and 70.6% of the elderly women rated their overall satisfaction with life as high and positive.

Medeiros (2012) carried out an inductive study using oral examinations and extensive forms, the same used by the SB Brasil 2010 project, in order to test the association between the outcome of endentulism/use and need for dental prostheses and socioeconomic data and access in adults and the elderly in Bayeux (Paraíba, João Pessoa), a municipality in the northeast of Brazil. The survey was carried out with a probabilistic sample of adults (n=64) and the elderly (n=22), according to criteria established by the World Health Organisation (WHO). The specific results for the elderly age group included 22 elderly people of both sexes and the prevalence of elderly people using upper prostheses was 50%, the use of lower prostheses was 7%, but 73% already needed upper prostheses and 91% lower prostheses. The results obtained in relation to risk factors for needing dentures were: age (OR=1.07), self-reported need for dental treatment (OR=32.02) and having gone to the dentist for the following reasons: tooth extraction (OR=5.58) and treatment (OR=14.69.). In conclusion, the prevalence of dental prostheses in the municipality is high, and the need for prostheses in the older population is significant.

A study carried out in Monte Negro (RO) by Xavier et al. (2011) assessed the need for prostheses in the municipality, which was co-related with the 2003 Brazilian Health Survey. In the elderly group, they found that 57.9 per cent needed upper total prostheses, with 33 per cent of the participants aged between 45 and 65. In the lower arch, the use of full dentures was 52.6 per cent and 21.43 per cent for the age group mentioned above.

Correa (2011) assessed the satisfaction and quality of prosthetic treatment carried out in the Dental Speciality Centres (DSC) of Greater Natal, including the municipalities of Natal, Macaíba, Paramirim and São Gonçalo do Amarante. The study was carried out between 2007 and 2009. A total of 149 users were examined and 233 total prostheses were made (148 upper and 85 lower). The result was satisfactory when it came to the upper prosthesis, with around 52.7% approval, while the lower prosthesis had 90.5% unsatisfactory cases. A total of 69.1% were satisfied with the prosthesis made at the DSC and 17.4% stopped using the prosthesis made at the DSC.

2.3 - Elderly Health in Amazonas

There are few records of epidemiological data on edentulism in the northern region of Brazil, especially in the state of Amazonas. In 2011, a study was published in the municipality of Manaus, Amazonas (AM) by Cardoso et al. (2007) . 807 elderly people with an average age of 69.2 years of both sexes were interviewed, with females predominating (69.12%). The index of decayed, missing and filled teeth (DMFT) was assessed. This study concludes that there were significant differences in the prevalence of edentulous people between the capitals of the state of Amazonas and the Northern region. In Manaus, the elderly wear more upper dentures than lower ones and women have more tooth loss than men.

Pontes (2009) selected two riverside communities in the municipality of Coari-AM in order to describe oral health conditions and analyse factors associated with the health-disease process. The two riverside communities chosen were selected according to their location: one should be closer to the municipality's headquarters (Isidoro Community) and the other more distant (Lauro Sodré Community). A cross-sectional study was carried out according to the WHO (World Health Organisation) criteria for epidemiological research into oral health. Individuals aged between 1 and 75 were selected. The OHIP questionnaire was administered to individuals over the age of 18.

14 in order to describe the oral impacts. It was noted that the high prevalence of periodontal disease and edentulism (in adults and the elderly) are not the most important problems for the riverside dwellers. The conditions that cause the most impact are related to toothache, which occurs without dental care and without palliative mediation, the presence of root remnants that need to be extracted and teeth with untreated caries. It reveals that the perception of river dwellers regarding the negative impacts caused by oral diseases has a different weight to the need for treatment of this population, since many do not have access to dental care due to the difficulty of river transport. The results of the qualitative analysis of the interviews revealed: the absence of a permanent dental service in the community; sporadic provision by means of health boats, with less occurrence of more distant community services; the high cost for river dwellers to go to the municipal headquarters (travelling by river is more common in this region); dental treatment focused on pain control, with the clinical outcome being exodontia. In view of the precarious access of river dwellers to oral health services, there is a notable need to implement wide-ranging health promotion measures, combined with a greater supply of services.

Beloni (2013) carried out a study to assess the level of life satisfaction of denture wearers at the Dental Polyclinic of the School of Health Science of the State University of Amazonas (UEA), using the OHIP-EDENT questionnaire, specific for edentulous people, and the visual analogue scale (VAS), and selected 39 adult patients of both genders rehabilitated with removable complete dentures (TP) or removable partial dentures (RP). Of the 39 patients selected, 32 took part in the study because they had no impediment. Of the 32 patients, 24 were female and eight were male. The age range was 34 to 63 years. Seventeen patients were rehabilitated with an upper full denture, one with a double full denture and eight with a removable partial denture. The results show that the type of prosthesis can influence the subjective parameters of patient satisfaction with rehabilitation and quality of life after oral rehabilitation with prostheses. Patients wearing complete dentures showed greater satisfaction with stability and masticatory function after rehabilitation.

Cardoso (2009), in his dissertation to characterise the oral health of elderly people living in Manaus/ Amazonas/ Brazil, carried out a population-based cross-sectional study in which 667 elderly people aged between 65 and 74 took part. Oral health was assessed based on psychological-social, physical and pain aspects using the GOHAI. The results obtained were: the use of dentures was more frequent in the upper arch (87.71%) than in the lower arch (52.92%), corroborated by the greater need for dentures in the lower arch (67.92%). The highest frequency of total prosthesis use for both arches was 79.1% and 36.73%, respectively. Of those interviewed, 42.88% needed upper full dentures and 33.01% needed lower removable partial dentures. Regarding self-assessment of oral health, 72.39% of the elderly rated it positively and only 10.26% rated it as bad/very bad. The frequency of positive evaluations remained for the appearance of teeth and gums, chewing and speech, with 66.31 to 75.79 per cent of the elderly rating themselves as good/optimally. Relationships with other people were reported to be unaffected by 86.51% of the elderly. Most of the elderly had a high self-assessment of their oral health, with a total score equal to or greater than 34 for 67.12% of the elderly, followed by 21.77% with a moderate rating and only 11.11% with a negative rating. Regarding the use and need for prostheses, both for the upper and lower arches, 75.56% and 75.67% respectively. Among the edentulous, 84.01% rated their oral health positively, 12.50% rated it as fair and only 3.49% as bad or very bad. For the dentate elderly, only 58.23% rated their oral health as good or excellent.

Cardoso (2010) carried out a population-based cross-sectional study with 667 individuals aged 65-74 in order to characterise the oral health conditions of elderly residents in the municipality of Manaus, Amazonas, according to gender. Interviews were conducted to ascertain demographic and socioeconomic information. The oral examination for caries, edentulism, use and need for prostheses was conducted in accordance with the WHO. The results obtained according to gender were mostly female, totalling 461 women and 206 men, with an average age of 69.2 years. The oral health results of the participants were described and the average number of teeth per individual was 4.1 +-5.7 and the prevalence of edentulism was 52.2%, in which only 3% of the elderly had 20 teeth or more. The use of upper and lower prostheses was observed in 79.2% and 37.1%, respectively. When comparing the sexes, it was noted that males had a lower rate of decayed, missing and filled teeth, more teeth and less edentulism. The use of upper and lower prostheses was higher in females, while the need for single or partial upper and lower prostheses was higher in the elderly.

A quantitative study comparing the living conditions and health of the elderly in the cities of Manaus and Porto Alegre carried out by Cauduro (2011) included 1,547 elderly people, 1,078 from the Porto Alegre Elderly Project and 469 from the Manaus Elderly Project. The study included individuals aged 60 or over of both sexes living in both states. The study is spread over 12 chapters and among them is a report on the health of the elderly in the two cities and when mentioning chewing difficulties, it was revealed that in Manaus 386 (82.7%) and Porto Alegre 812 (75.3%) had no chewing difficulties. Also in the study, in relation to the use of dental prostheses, there is a need highlighted by the elderly where in Manaus 75 (16.1%) and Porto Alegre 75 (16.1%) the elderly use dental prostheses. An important piece of information about the diet of the elderly revealed in the study is the number of meals eaten during the day, and the option most cited by the elderly in both cities was "three times a day", in which Manaus 264 (56.4%) and Porto Alegre 498 (46.2%). Next up in both Manaus and Porto Alegre were "four" 127 (27.1%) and 313 (29.0%); "five" 33 (7.1%) and 129 (12.0%); "two" 31 (6.6%) and 107 (9.9%); and "one" 8 (1.7%) and 107 (9.9%), respectively.

2.4 - Evaluation of Satisfaction with Total Prosthesis

Not only does not having teeth affect chewing, but it also has an impact on facial appearance, because over time cheeks, lips and chin become more prominent, nose droops and bite collapses, all of which affect the patient's self-esteem. Pesqueiro (2005) assessed the psychological aspects of 130 patients of both sexes and concluded in this study that wearing a satisfactory prosthesis is important for self-esteem and commented that wearing a prosthesis influences social relationships, but is not fundamental. Prostheses don't influence emotional life, but when it comes to quality, they can have a negative influence, also affecting patients' sex lives.

Ramos et al. (2001) observed that the main problems presented by patients using complete dentures are: lack of stability and retention, unsatisfactory aesthetics, low masticatory efficiency and altered vertical occlusion dimension. The basal area, where the base of the prosthesis will be adapted, which is made up of bone, mucosa and submucosa, should be taken into consideration in an attempt to make the prosthesis as comfortable as possible for the patient.

Turano and Turano (2002) say that when there are flat rims, it is difficult to obtain a retentive and stable total prosthesis. This is why the preservation of bone tissue is of paramount importance, considering that success is achieved when the bone base remains intact.

Barbosa et al. (2006) state that the installation of complete dentures must be carried out carefully by the professional, observing retention, stability, support, occlusion, compression area, stretch and phonetics.

Cabrini et al (2008) carried out a study with 166 patients whose inclusion criteria were edentulous patients and users of bi-maxillary total prostheses, in which the time of use was analysed in terms of the general quality of the prostheses. A total of 112 female and 54 male patients took part in the study, with a mean age of 65.3 years. The results showed that 73 patients had been wearing their prostheses for less than five years, 23 for between 5 and 10 years and 70 for more than 10 years. When asked about quality, 52 patients considered it good, 54 fair and 59 poor. It was concluded that time has an influence on the overall quality of complete dentures, as does the arrangement of anterior teeth, the interocclusal distance, occlusal articulation and edge extension of mandibular complete dentures are strongly influenced by time of use, unlike stability and retention.

Assunção et al. (2004) reported that for total dentures to fit properly, the para-prosthetic anatomical structures must be respected so that there is stability and retention, providing comfort and durability. Knowledge of the anatomy is fundamental for patient satisfaction.

Lopes (2010) analysed and compared the masticatory capacity of dentate and edentulous patients using various prostheses. The clinical records and questionnaires before and after prosthetic rehabilitation were analysed to ascertain the level of masticatory capacity, using scores from 0-1-2 for different types of food (soft, solid and hard). The majority were women aged between 60 and 69. From the data, it was concluded that there is a masticatory difference between the different foods. Another result was that the greater the stability of the prosthesis, the greater the patient's chewing efficiency and sensitivity during food processing.

Steca (2007) assessed the level of satisfaction, retention and stability of conventional complete dentures at the Juiz de Fora School of Medical and Health Sciences. Twelve patients were selected as they met the necessary requirements for the study, according to the inclusion criteria: total edentulous patients who wore upper and lower total prostheses (the pair). The patients underwent an anamnesis to check their general health. The results showed that the patients were satisfied with their new complete dentures in terms of aesthetics, increasing positivity and emotional attitude. The majority felt comfortable. There was 100% satisfaction with retention and stability, but three patients (27%) were dissatisfied with the lower prostheses.

Goiato et al. (2012), in their study, selected 60 patients who had been wearing bimaxillary complete dentures for more than 5 years to assess the quality of life and examine the sensation of complete denture wearers before and after the insertion of new dentures. The patients were assessed in 2011, first in April and again in June, after three months of use with the new prosthesis. The authors reported that after rehabilitation, the patients showed acceptance, satisfaction, quality of life, improved chewing and speech, comfort, retention and stability of the new prosthesis. It was concluded that total denture rehabilitation was effective in terms of quality of life and patient perception.

Gabardo et al (2013) carried out a literature review using the Oral Health Impact Profile (OHIP) instrument to measure the impact of oral health in its different forms. They selected 20 articles with a cross-sectional design, according to the inclusion criteria adopted, and identified that the worst self-perception of oral health is associated with unfavourable social, economic, demographic, psychosocial and behavioural factors, as well as poor clinical oral conditions. They concluded that the use of the OHIP instrument is important in helping to clarify oral health needs and in drawing up strategies to control/reduce diseases and promote oral health with a positive impact on quality of life.

The general objective was to assess the level of satisfaction of patients treated at the teaching dental clinic of the Universidade Paulista -UNIP Manaus campus, for the manufacture of complete dentures.

The specific objectives were: to compare the old total prosthesis with the new one; to assess the degree of patient satisfaction in relation to the aesthetics and functionality of the new total prosthesis; to assess patient comfort with the prosthesis in relation to speech and chewing; to assess retention and stability of the prosthesis; and proservation after six months.

The hypothesis was in relation to the care offered to patients who seek care at the Universidade Paulista - Manaus itself, knowing how they found out and what made them seek care, evaluating the old prosthesis with the new one, using the OHIP-14 (Oral Health Impact Profile-Short From) questionnaire, made up of seven topics with two questions each, where patients reveal their answers according to the response options. The questionnaire was administered twice, once with the old prosthesis and once after six months of use.

Based on the importance of total prostheses in the quality of life of edentulous patients, this study was carried out at the total prosthesis clinic at the Universidade Paulista - Manaus campus. The aim was to analyse the profile of the patients, the reason for their edentulism, their search for the service at a university and their satisfaction with receiving the prosthesis within a week and after six months. It was important to know the profile of the patients who sought the service, their satisfaction and their return after six months to assess whether their use was satisfactory or not.

Munoz (2011) mentions that one of the treatment options for tooth replacement, in the case of edentulism, would be the use of a mucosupported total prosthesis, which would restore the user's lost functions such as aesthetics, comfort, health, phonetics, posture and stomach balance.

The patient considers the total prosthesis to be satisfactory when it restores aesthetics, function and phonetics, and for the professional, satisfaction comes from the fact that the patient leaves the office happy with an improved quality of life.

CHAPTER 3

METHOD

This study was carried out in the city of Manaus (AM), at the Faculty of Dentistry of Universidade Paulista - UNIP, after approval by the Ethics Committee, whose opinion number 142.042 was approved, as shown in Annex 1.

The sample consisted of twelve patients who came to the mucous-supported total prosthesis clinic, a subject that is part of the curriculum for 3rd/4th year undergraduates at the school.

After the patients had read and signed the Informed Consent Form (ICF), Appendix 2. The questionnaires were administered and all accepted voluntary participation in this study.

The questionnaire used to ascertain the satisfaction and quality of the prostheses was the OHIP-14 (Oral Health Impact Profile-Short From), which has been translated and adapted for Brazil. It is currently used as the main study. The original Australian version of the OHIP, made up of 49 items, is a questionnaire used worldwide when it comes to patient satisfaction, which is the aim of this study. The OHIP-14 questionnaire is made up of seven topics, each consisting of two questions, limited to function, physical pain, psychological discomfort, physical inability, psychological inability and functional limitation. Answers are given according to a coded scale: 1 = never, 2 = almost never, 3 = sometimes, 4 = fairly often and 5 = very often. The higher the value given by the interviewee, the worse the self-perception of the impact. The interviewer read out the questions and the patients answered according to the options and their own opinion (listed above from 1 to 5), everyone was free to make any observations during the interviews as well as during the follow-up. The patients returned to answer the same OHIP-14 questionnaire again, and a new clinical examination was carried out to assess the oral cavity as well as the use of prostheses. During these months, the patients were free to comment on the months of use of the removable total prosthesis.

At the first moment of the interview, they answered the time and reason for losing their teeth, as well as the questions: what changed in your life when you lost your teeth? Why did you choose to wear full dentures? What are your expectations of wearing a new full denture?

The data obtained during the interviews was transferred to Microsoft Office Excel 2007, and also Microsoft Office Word 2007 to make the tables. The statistical tests used were the Mann-Whitney U-test for the age range of the patients and the Kappa test for the occurrence of prostheses.

The second stage was the follow-up period to monitor the evolution of the patient's clinical state of oral health and general health. Six months after the prostheses were delivered, the patient was scheduled to return for a repeat of the OHIP-14 questionnaire and an assessment of the oral cavity, at the university itself, according to each patient's availability.

CHAPTER 4

RESULTS

Of the patients interviewed, nine were female and three were male, living in the city of Manaus, AM. Their average age was 51.58 years, which is considered young, as shown in Table 1. As for place of birth, ten were from the interior of Amazonas, one from Manaus and one from Campina Grande (PB).

TABLE 1 - AGE OF PATIENTS

AGE	NUMBER OF PATIENTS	PERCENTAGE
Under 64	8	66,6%
65-70 years old	3	25,0%
From 71-75 years old	1	08,3%
From 76-80 years old	0	0%
Over 81 years old	0	0%
TOTAL	12	100%

Regarding the indication of the prostheses to be made, they could be upper, lower or a pair (upper + lower). Five upper prostheses and seven lower prostheses were made. When asked about the reason for tooth loss, six patients said it was due to caries, one due to periodontal problems and five reported other reasons (such as: lack of access to the dentist, thought it was nice to have to wear dentures, extracted teeth at a young age). As shown in the table below:

Table 2 - Etiology of Edentulism

Reasons	Numbers	Percentage
Caries	6	50,0%
Periodontics	1	08,3%
Others	5	41,6%
Total	12	100%

Patients were asked what changed when they lost their teeth. The answers included:

eating, taste, chewing, self-esteem, fear of the prosthesis falling out and bad odour. There was a special case of a patient who commented that kissing wasn't the same either. He lost his teeth around the age of 18, because he thought it was beautiful to wear dentures, and during the treatment he had intended to have an implant (overdenture), in another course also in the city of Manaus, which ended up not happening.

When the question was related to changing the prosthesis for a new one, many of the answers were related to aesthetics, retention and stability, and quality of life.

The OHIP-14 questionnaire was then administered. In this questionnaire, the answers were objective and if there was any need to supplement the answer to a question, the patients could do so.

TABLE 4: - First Interview - OHIP-14 Questionnaire

	Never (1)	Almost never (2)	Sometimes (3)	Fair frequency (4)	Very frequent (5)
Functional limitation:					
1. Speak	6 (50.0)	0 (0.0)	5 (41.6)	1 (8.3)	0 (0.0)
2. Taste	8 (66.6)	1 (8.3)	2 (16.6)	0 (0.0)	1 (8.3)
Physical pain:					
3. Severe pain	7 (58.3)	1 (8.3)	2 (16.6)	1 (8.3)	1 (8.3)
4. Uncomfortable eating	3 (25.0)	3 (25.0)	2 (16.6)	1 (8.3)	3 (25.0)
Psychological discomfort					
5. Constrained	8 (66.6)	1 (8.3)	1 (8.3)	2 (16.6)	0 (0.0)
6. Tension	7 (58.3)	1 (8.3)	3 (25.0)	1 (8.3)	0 (0.0)
Physical Inability					
7. Unsatisfactory diet	7 (58.3)	0 (0.0)	5 (41.6)	0 (0.0)	0 (0.0)
8. Interrupting the power supply	8 (66.6)	1 (8.3)	1 (8.3)	2 (16.6)	0 (0.0)
Psychological Inability:					
9. Relax	9 (75.0)	1 (8.3)	0 (0.0)	0 (0.0)	2 (16.6)
10. Embarrassed	8 (66.6)	0 (0.0)	3 (25.0)	1 (8.3)	0 (0.0)
Social Inability:					
11. Angry	11(91.6)	1 (8.3)	0 (0.0)	0 (0.0)	0 (0.0)
12. Daily tasks	10(83.3)	1 (8.3)	1 (8.3)	0 (0.0)	0 (0.0)
Functional Limitation:					
13. Less satisfaction with life	10(83.3)	1 (8.3)	0 (0.0)	1 (8.3)	0 (0.0)
14. Totally incapable	9 (75.0)	1 (8.3)	1 (8.3)	1 (8.3)	0 (0.0)

In December 2011, the prostheses were installed and the patients were given a week to adapt. After this period, all patients had to return for a reassessment of the prosthesis in the oral cavity. If any discomfort was reported, the patients were instructed to discontinue use and on their return they would be adapted according to each patient's needs.

On returning after a week's use, the changes were remarkable. Some of the women were wearing make-up and loose hair, which they hadn't done before. On entering the clinic, one of the patients was more confident and spoke up, as he had been quite shy during the prosthesis fitting period. Both sexes showed an improvement in self-esteem.

Only one patient did not return after the installation of the new prosthesis. Of those who did return, eight patients reported not having felt any discomfort in relation to their prosthesis. Two experienced pain and one had inflammatory fibrous hyperplasia caused by premature contact. With the appropriate observations, adjustments were made and the patients were discharged and scheduled to return the following week if the discomfort returned. If they didn't, they wouldn't return, which meant that the prosthesis was favourable for use in the users' view.

The follow-up took place after six months, when the patients were contacted again for a return visit, taking into account the best time for each patient. On this return visit, all the patients underwent a clinical examination to check for any lesions caused by the use of the prosthesis. No lesions were recorded in any of the patients, and the prostheses were in a favourable state of use. The patient who reported not being satisfied was referred to the clinic to have a new prosthesis made, but he did not return to the university.

TABLE 4: AFTER 6 MONTHS OF USE - Second Interview. OHIP Questionnaire 14

	Never (1)	Almost never (2)	Sometimes (3)	Fair frequency (4)	Very frequent (5)
Functional limitation: 1. Speech	9 (75.0)	2 (16.6)	1 (8.3)	0 (0.0)	0 (0.0)
2. Taste	10 (83.3)	2 (16.6)	0 (0.0)	0 (0.0)	0 (0.0)
Physical pain:					
3. Severe pain	9 (75.0)	3 (25.0)	0 (0.0)	0 (0.0)	0 (0.0)
4. Uncomfortable eating	5 (41.6)	3 (25.0)	3 (25.0)	1 (8.3)	0 (0.0)
Psychological discomfort:					
5. Constrained	10 (83.3)	1 (8.3)	1 (8.3)	0 (0.0)	0 (0.0)
6. Tension	10 (83.3)	2 (16.6)	0 (0.0)	0 (0.0)	0 (0.0)
Physical inability:					
7. Unsatisfactory diet	7 (58.3)	4 (33.3)	1 (8.3)	0 (0.0)	0 (0.0)
8. Interrupting the power supply	8 (66.6)	3 (25.0)	0 (0.0)	1 (8.3)	0 (0.0)
Psychological Inability:					
9. Relax	9 (75.0)	2 (16.6)	1 (8.3)	0 (0.0)	0 (0.0)
10. Embarrassed	8 (66.6)	3 (25.0)	1 (8.3)	0 (0.0)	0 (0.0)

Social Inability:					
11. Angry	11 (91.6)	0 (0.0)	1 (8.3)	0 (0.0)	0 (0.0)
12. Daily tasks	11 (91.6)	1 (8.3)	0 (0.0)	0 (0.0)	0 (0.0)
Functional Limitation:					
13. Less satisfaction with life	11 (91.6)	1 (8.3)	0 (0.0)	0 (0.0)	0 (0.0)
14. Totally incapable	11 (91.6)	1 (8.3)	0 (0.0)	0 (0.0)	0 (0.0)

When they returned for the second interview, according to the data in Table 5, the patients were generally satisfied. The prosthesis had good stability and retention. There was an improvement in self-esteem, but when asked about chewing, two patients reported that they felt uncomfortable chewing regional foods such as Uarini flour, tapioca flour and even the fish itself, as well as one who commented that he liked eating chicken bones because the prosthesis loses stability and moves out of position.

The statistical data will be organised according to the questions on each topic of the OHIP-14 questionnaire, analysing before and after the new prosthesis. According to the Kappa statistical test for prosthesis events before and after the installation of the new prosthesis. Regarding functional limitations in terms of speech, the value was $p=0.1030$ and $\alpha=5\%$ and taste, the value was $p=0.1182$ and $\alpha=5\%$. Regarding physical pain, the value for severe pain was $p=0.1932$ and $\alpha=5\%$ and discomfort when eating was $p=0.1932$ and $\alpha=5\%$. Psychological discomfort in the embarrassment requirement had a value of $p=0.1729$ and $\alpha=5\%$ and tension had a value of $p=0.0889$ and $\alpha=5\%$. Physical inability when asked about unsatisfactory diet was $p=0.5000$ and $\alpha=5\%$ and interrupted eating $p=0.5000$ and $\alpha=5\%$. Psychological inability to relax and being embarrassed had a value of $p=0.5000$ and $\alpha=5\%$. Social inability to get angry was $p=0.2685$ and $\alpha=5\%$. and daily tasks was $p=0.2685$ and $\alpha=5\%$. Physical limitation in the fact that they felt less satisfied with life was $p=0.2685$ and $\alpha=5\%$ and totally incapable was $p=0.1367$ and $\alpha=5\%$. Indicating both before the new prosthesis and after the new prosthesis, the majority of interviewees did not report that there were no changes in relation to their answers.

CHAPTER 5

DISCUSSION

This study assessed the profile of the patients treated at the Total Prosthesis Clinic of the Dentistry Clinic of the UNIP-AM teaching institution, in which there was a prevalence of females and an average age of 51.58 years. The Mann-Whitney U-test used as statistical data revealed that there was no statistically significant difference between the ages of the male and female interviewees, according to the p-value of 0.2294 and $\alpha = 5\%$.

Hilgenberg (2011) carried out a study on phonetics in patients with dentures, citing that a dental procedure should always combine aesthetics, masticatory function (chewing and swallowing), oral functions, neuromuscular balance and phonetics. The patient's adaptation time with the prosthesis lasts around six to eight months. A variant in adaptation time is the tongue. The larger the patient's tongue, the more difficult it is to adapt. The positioning of the teeth and the shape of the palate are the two variants that make adaptation possible. At the end of his study, he mentioned that the dental surgeon should be aware of phonetic evaluation, which should be carried out before starting treatment, or during the provisional phase, or even during the wax teeth test. The conscientious professional stands out from the rest.

In this study, the patients were evaluated after six months of using the new prosthesis, and the following were observed: quality of life, self-esteem, improved social interaction for those who felt their prosthesis was comfortable and favourable to use.

Menezes (2007) cites the main vocal complaints and symptoms reported by the elderly and which can alter vocal quality, such as hoarseness and aphonia, tiredness associated with voice production, efforts to improve vocal projection, breathiness, lack of vocal modulation, shaky voice, difficulty controlling vocal intensity, pain in the shoulder girdle region and a burning sensation or foreign body in the larynx. Tooth loss and ill-fitting dentures create difficulties in articulation, aggravated by decreased saliva and reduced tone in the orofacial muscles. Modifications to the supraglottic vocal tract include growth of the facial skeleton, hypertrophy of the tongue musculature, loss of teeth, weakening of the pharyngeal musculature and restricted movement of the temperomandibular joint.

Matiello (2005) reports that retention and stability are the most frequent needs of patients and this has led to various techniques and materials being researched for their comfort. The difficulty in satisfaction is when it comes to re-establishing masticatory function, when compared to dentists. In addition, the use of hard food causes the most problems for denture wearers, who do not feel satisfied with soft food alone.

A particular case cited in this study by the patients themselves is the food that accompanies meals in the Amazonas region, where the native diet is based on manioc flour, tapioca flour, fish of varying sizes and hardness, forming part of the daily meal of the natives, and one of the foods that the denture wearer has difficulty chewing, causing discomfort in chewing and causing a reduction in the temperature of the food, because in some cases the palate is sealed.

Pinelli et. al (2004) say in their study that it often happens that the criteria for a dentist to be considered excellent may be that the patient is not so satisfied, because they have a different perspective, and satisfaction is important for both sides, for the treatment itself. In our study, this perception was very clear, with the elderly reporting on their daily diet, where they stop eating manioc flour, bite into chicken bones, tapioca beans, where they themselves miss it or feel insecure, because they are hard foods and vary in size, which loses the retention and stability of the prosthesis.

The sensory perception of the elderly in relation to food is the result of a series of factors that involve ageing, such as medication that alters tasting and poor hygiene (Manet, 1998; Monteiro, 2009). In our study, it was clear that this perception was reported by the elderly as having difficulty due to their own lost oral physiology, the use of medication and an incomplete diet.

Muniz (2011) reported in his study that the success of prosthetics requires a relationship between the patient and the professional, where both are important for user satisfaction. The patient must have the opportunity to express their feelings about the appearance of their teeth or the appearance of the prosthesis. The professional must have the correct mastery of materials and technique, and transmit safety during the service.

In our study, patient satisfaction was assessed using the OHIP-14 questionnaire. This questionnaire asks specific questions about the changes patients perceive in their oral cavity. As well as answering the objective questions, patients could also give their opinion on the treatment they had received, leaving them free to complete the answers on the questionnaire itself. Only one patient was dissatisfied with the treatment, while the other patients who returned after the stipulated time were satisfied with their prostheses and had a better quality of life. This data could only be collected once the patients were invited to take part in this evaluation of the quality of the service provided by UNIP - Manaus campus, and any doubts they had were clarified.

Pesqueiro (2005) says that the quality of oral health plays an important role in the lives of the elderly. When it is compromised, it negatively affects nutritional levels, physical and mental well-being and can diminish the enjoyment of a social life. Concluding that prostheses influence affective life and there is no negative interference from their use in affective life (78%), but quality can be important in affective relationships (79.3%).

In our study, we observed that there was an improvement in all the topics that are part of the OHIP-14 questionnaire, and we noted from the patients' responses that it is possible to improve their functional limitations and psychosocial discomfort.

Serman et. al (2003) observed the prevalence of signs and symptoms of Mandibular Temperament Dysfunction in patients wearing full dentures compared to denture wearers. The sample included 100 patients equally divided into two groups. Group I consisted of double denture wearers and Group II of denture patients. Both groups answered a questionnaire with 10 questions relating to TMD (temporomandibular dysfunction), and group one answered a further four questions relating to dentures. The study concluded that the rate of TMD is higher in patients with dentures, with no specific relationship to the denture. And the prevalence of TMD is higher in women in both groups. In our study, this data was evaluated. When comparing the results of the first consultation in table 4, 41.5% of the patients (1,2,3,4) felt pain when wearing the old prosthesis and 75% (1,2,3,4) felt some discomfort and with the new prosthesis after 6 months 25% almost never (2) felt strong pain and 58.3% (1,2,3) felt some discomfort when chewing.

Cavalcante (2004), in an epidemiological survey of bus terminals in the city of Curitiba, where a group of 60 researchers used a questionnaire formulated by the Centre for the Diagnosis and Treatment of the Tempero-Mandibular Joint and Dento-Facial Alterations at the Tuiuti University of Paraná, interviewed 5,186 people, of whom 1,134 (21.86%) were totally edentulous and of these around 450 (40%) had orofacial pain. It is assumed that total edentulous patients present morphological and functional alterations to the stomatognathic system, which may be contributing factors to the onset of orofacial pain, such as parafunctional habits, occlusal alterations, prosthesis instability, iatrogenic problems and worsening of stomatognathic system functions (swallowing, chewing, phonation and breathing). Based on these assumptions, it is understood that with the correct rehabilitation of these patients, after proper diagnosis, planning and treatment in accordance with scientific criteria, it is possible to aim for remission of their symptoms.

Silva et al (2010) report that tooth loss has the greatest impact on feeling ashamed, where the user reports embarrassment when smiling, especially when missing front teeth. When comparing tables (3 and 4) in relation to embarrassment, it can be seen that there was no change in the patients' responses, citing that there is no discomfort because it is a prosthesis, apart from the insecurity that the prosthesis may fall off, which usually happens when speaking.

Silva et al (2006) assessed the overall satisfaction of 17 women, all over the age of 60, who sought services to have a new prosthesis made at the Total Prosthesis Clinic of the Piracicaba School of Dentistry. The GOHAI questionnaire and the Cantril Self-Assessment scale were used to measure overall life satisfaction. 59.9 per cent rated their oral health as low and 70.6 per cent rated their overall life satisfaction as high and positive. The authors concluded that although patients reported unsatisfactory oral health, this did not interfere with high global life satisfaction.

Pontes (2009), in seeking to understand quality of life, cites that it is understood as the degree to which a person appreciates the important possibilities of life. It is multidirectional and depends on 1. factors external to the individual (social, cultural, economic and political); 2. state of health and health related to quality of life (symptoms, functional state and components of health perception); 3. factors internal to individuals (biological, lifestyle, health behaviour, personality and values). When mentioning oral diseases, he emphasises that most of them are not fatal, but lead to significant morbidity and result in physical, social and psychological consequences that affect quality of life. The most commonly cited are pain, speech difficulties, chewing ability, taste and the appearance of teeth.

Guimarães et. al (2013) report that social inability is the dimension that has the least impact on the quality of life of elderly users of complete dentures. When compared with the present study, we found that 91.6% never felt irritated with other people and 83.3% felt unable to carry out daily activities, both related to the mouth, teeth and dentures and 91.6% for both questions in the second consultation. Compared to the other questions, the relationship between irritability and carrying out tasks was not affected by the use of dentures.

CHAPTER 6

FINAL CONSIDERATIONS

In this study, we came to the following conclusions:

O The prevalent gender among the patients who took part in the study was female;

- The predominant age group was patients under 64;
- Among the motivations for using dentures are aesthetics, phonetics and patient comfort;
- Edentulism, the absence of teeth, has unfavourable emotional consequences for the patient;
- Compared to the two consultations, there were improvements reported in the second interview, proservation, mainly in functional limitation, psychological discomfort, social inability and physical limitation, demonstrating greater importance in rehabilitation, with an improvement in retention and stability and self-confidence;
- The main types of discomfort reported were when questioned about physical and psychological inability, which was justified because it was considered less relevant;
- The statistical tests showed no change in the answers, and the changes were considered random.

In the biopsychosocial context of the individual, primary prevention is necessary as a fundamental strategy for the health of the elderly and the present work takes this perspective with the return after its delivery and follow-up after six months to identify what the changes were in relation to the stimulated time.

Good treatment requires a positive relationship between the patient and the professional, where both must be in tune with each other, recognising the patient's profile and giving them the opportunity to set out their expectations. The return of stomatognathic function is favourable in terms of satisfaction and quality of life, as is the improvement in the patient's nutritional diet. When replaced, the benefit generated by the replacement is noticeable. The state needs to pay more attention to this service, since as quality of life increases, so does the demand from elderly patients who need prostheses and a quality service.

In order to increase life expectancy and improve the quality of life of the elderly, greater attention needs to be paid to this group, as the information described in this study contributes to the implementation of new public and private health policies.

CHAPTER 7

BIBLIOGRAPHICAL REFERENCES

ASSUNÇÃO, W. et al.Para-Prosthetic Anatomy: Importance in Total Prosthesis. Revista Odontológica de Araçatuba, n.1, v.25, p. 57-64.2004,

BARBOSA,D.et al. Installation of complete dentures: a review.**Revista de** Odontologia da UNESP.; n. 35, v.1, p. 53-60, 2006.

BELONI, W. B.; VALE, H. F.; TAKAHASI, J. M. F. K. Evaluation of the degree of satisfaction and quality of life of denture wearers. RFO, Passo Fundo, v.08, n.2, PP. 160-164. Available at:< http://revodonto.bvsalud.org/scielo.php?script=sci arttext&pid=S1413-40122013000200006&lng=pt >. Accessed on: 10 May 2018.

BOMFIM, I. P. R. et al. Prevalence of Oral Mucosa Lesions in Patients with Dentures. Pesquisa Brasileira em Odontopediatria e Clínica Integrada. Red de Revista Científicas de América Latina y el Caribe, Espana y Portugal. 2008. Disponívelem :< http://www.redalyc.org/html/637/63711702019/ >. Accessed on 10 May , 2018.

BRAZIL. Ministry of Health. SB Brasil 2003 Project: oral health conditions of the Brazilian population 2002-2003: Main Results. Brasília: Ministry of Health; 2004.

Brazil. Ministry of Health. Department of Primary Health Care. Department of Primary Care. Technical manual for the fabrication of complete dentures using the

microwave polymerisation / Ministry of Health. Secretary of Health Care. Department of

Primary Care. - Brasília: Ministry of Health, 2012.

BRAZIL, Ministry of Health. SB Brasil 2010 Project SBBrasil 2010 Project: National Oral Health Survey: Main Results. Brasília: Ministry of Health; 2011.

BRITO, M. C. C.; FREITAS, C. A. S. L.; MESQUITA, K. O.; LIMA, G. K. Population ageing and the challenges for public health: an analysis of scientific production. Revista Kaíros Gerontologia, 16 (3), pp 161-178. Sao Paulo (SP), Brazil. Available at :< https://revistas.pucsp.br/index.php/kairos/article/view/18552 > Accessed on:20, April.

BRUNETTI, R. F; MONTENEGRO, F. L; MANETTA, C. E. Questions and answers about dental care for the elderly. Available at:<http://portaldoenvelhecimento.org.br/noticias/odontogeriatria/perguntas-e-answers-about-dental-care-for-the-elderly.html> Accessed on: 25 August 2012.

CABRINI, J.et al. Wearing time and the quality of complete dentures - a critical analysis.Faculdade de Odontologia de Araraquara - UNESP.São Paulo, 2008.

CARDOSO, E. et al. Oral health status of elderly residents in the municipality of Manaus, Amazonas: estimates by gender. Rev Bras Epidemiol; 14(1): 13140. 2011.

CHAIMOWICZ, F. et al. Saúde do Idoso. 2ª Edition: Belo Horizonte: NESCON UFMG, 2013.

COLUSSI, C. F.; FREITAS, S. F. T. Aspectos epidemiológicos da saúde bucal do idoso no Brasil. Cadernos de Saúde Pública, Rio de Janeiro, volume there, number 05, 02 March 2013. Available at:< https://www.scielosp.org/scielo.php?pid=S0102-311X2002000500024&script=sci arttext&tlng=es >. Accessed on:06, May, 2018.

COSTA, A.P. S. Satisfaction of users and quality of prosthetic treatments carried out in the Dental Speciality Centres of Greater Natal -RN.(Master's degree in Preventive and Social Dentistry) Federal University of Rio Grande do Norte, 2011.

DAWALIBI, N. W.; ANACLETO, G. M. C.; WITTER, C.; GOULART, R. M. M.; AQUINO, R. C. Ageing and quality of life: an analysis of SciELO scientific production. Estudos de Psicilogia. Campinas - São Paulo. 30(3) ; July-September.

ETTINGER, R. L. Changing dietary patterns with changing dentition: How do peoplecope? Special Care in Dentistry. Chicago, v.18, p.33-39. Jan./Feb. 1998.

FRAZAO, P.; ANTUNES, J. L. F.; NARVAI, P. C. Early tooth loss in adults aged 35 to 44 years. State of São Paulo, Brazil, 1998. Rev. Bras. Epidemiol. Vol. 6, No. 1, p. 50-51, 2003.

FURTADO, D. G.; FORTE, F. D. S.; LEITE, D. F. B. M. Uso e Necessidade de Prótese em Idosos: Reflexos na Qualidade de Vida. Revista Brasileira de Ciências da Saúde. volume 15, number 2, pages 183-190, 2011. Paraíba. João Pessoa.

G1, SÃO PAULO.Brazilians are born with life expectancy of 74 years and 29 days, says IBGE. available at:<http://g1. globo.com/brasil/noticia/2012/11/brasileiro-nasce-com-esperanca-de-vida-de-74-anos-e-29-dias-diz-ibge.html>. Accessed on: 11 January 2013.

GABARDO, M. C. L.; MOYSÉS, S. T.; MOYSÉS, S. J. Perception of oral health according to the Oral Health Impact Profile (OHIP) and associated factors: systematic review. Revista Panamericana de Salud Pública, volume 33, number 6, page 439-445, 2013.

GOIATO, M. et al.Quality of life and stimulus perception in patients' rehabilitated with complete denture. Journal of Oral Rehabilitation, v, 39, i. 6, p. 438-445, June 2012.

GUIMARÃES, M. B.et al. Impacto do uso de prótese dentaria totais na qualidade de vida de prótese dentarias totais na qualidade de vida de idosos. Brazilian Journal of Quality of Life. Ponta Grossa- PR. v. 05, n. 01,pg, 31-38, jan/mar 2013.

HILGENBERG, P. B.; PORTO, V. C. Phonetic Evaluation in Patients with Dentures. RGO-revista gaúcha odontol. Porto alegre. v. 59, suplemento 0, p. 75-79, jan/jun, 2011.

LOPES, C. C. R. Sensory analysis of chewing ability. 2010. 37 f. Monograph (Specialising in Implant Dentistry) - FAISA-CIODONTO, Rio de Janeiro, 2010.

LUCENA, S. C. **Functional assessment of dentures and patient satisfaction : correlation with masticatory performance and swallowing threshold**. University of Campinas. Piracicaba School of Dentistry 2010.

MANETTA, C.; BRUNETTI, R.. MONTENEGRO, F. Interactions between medicine and dentistry in the elderly - part I. Revista Atualidades em Geriatria(Soriak),v.3,n.20,p.5-13,Dec. 1998 .

MARTINS, A. M. E. B.; BARRETO, S. M.; PORDEUS, I. A. Characteristics associated with the use of dental services among dentate and edentate elderly in Southeast Brazil: SB Brasil Project. Caderno de Saúde Pública, volume 24, number 1, pages 81-92. June 2008. Rio de Janeiro. Available at:< http://www.scielo.br/scielo.php?pid=S0102-311X2008000100008&script=sci abstract&tlng=en >. Accessed on: 06, May, 2018.

MARUCH. A. et al. Impact of removable complete dentures on the quality of life of elderly people in social groups in Belo Horizonte - MG. Arquivos em Odontologia. v. 45, n° 02. April/June 2009.

MATIELLO, M. N.; SARTORI, I. A. M.; LOPES, J. F. S. Comparative analysis of the masticatory skills of dentate and edentulous patients rehabilitated with complete dentures. Salusvita, Bauru, v. 24, n. 3, p. 359-375, 2005.

MELLO, A. L. S. F.; ERDMAM, A. L.; CAETANO, J. C. Oral Health of the Elderly: Towards an Inclusive Policy. Texto Contexto Enferm, volume 17, number 4, pages 696-704, Oct-Dec 2008. Florianópolis. Available at: < http://www.scielo.br/pdf/tce/v17n4/10.pdf>. Accessed on 06 May 2018.

MENEZES, L. N.; VICENTE, L. C. C. Vocal ageing in institutionalised elderly people. Revista CEFAC, São Paulo , V.9, N.1, 90-8, Jan-Mar 2007.

MONTEIRO, M. A. M. Sensory Perception of Food in the Elderly. Revista Espaço para a Saúde, Londrina- Paraná, v. 10, n. 2, p. 34-42, jun. 2009.

MUNOZ, E. F. G.; ABREU, C. W. Factors influencing patient satisfaction with conventional complete dentures. HU Revista, Juiz de Fora, v. 37, n. 4, p. 413-419, Oct/Dec, 2011.

PESQUERO, A. C. B. Use of complete dentures by the elderly: psychological aspects. 2005. 55 pages Dissertation (Master's in Psychology) - Catholic University of Goiás. Goiânia, 2005.

PINELLI L, A. P. et al. Patient's Satisfaction with Fixed Partial Denture. Rev. Odontol. UNESP. 2004; 33 (2): 87-93.

PINTO, G. V. Saúde bucal coletiva. 4. ed. São Paulo: Santos, 2000
RAMOS, J. P. et al. Satisfaction of patients with complete dentures. JOFA, V.1, N.1, São Paulo, 2001.

SERMAN, R. J. et al. Prevalence of temporomandibular dysfunction in patients with double complete dentures. Jornal Brasileiro de Oclusão, Curitiba, v.3, n.10, p.141-144, Apr./Jun. 2003.

SHERMAN, H. Denture insertion. Dent Clin North Am; 21: 339-57. 1977

SIQUEIRA, A. F. C. et al. Masticatory ability, quality of life and satisfaction in Mandibular overdenture and removable partial denture wearers. Scientific Horizonavailable at   : <http://www.seer.ufu.br/index.php/horizontecientifico/issue/view/315>. Accessed on: 18 Oct, 2012.

STECCA, E. Evaluation of the Degree of Satisfaction, Retention and Stability of Conventional Full Dentures. 2007. 133 f. (Postgraduate dissertation in dentistry) - Veiga de Almeida University. Rio de Janeiro, 2007.

SILVA E. F. A.; SOUSA M. L. R. Self-perception of Oral Health and Satisfaction with Life in Elderly Women Wearing Full Dentures. Revista de Odontologia da Universidade Cidade de São Paulo. n.18, v.1, pg. 61-65 jan-abr; 2006.

SILVA, M. E. S.; VILLAÇA, E. L.; MAGALHÃES, C. S.; FERREIRA, E. F. Impact of tooth loss on quality of life. Ciênc. Saúde coletiva. Rio de Janeiro, v.15 n.3, May 2010.

SILVA, M. E. S.; MAGALHAES, C. S.; FERREIRA, E. F. Tooth loss and the expectation of prosthetic replacement: a qualitative study. Ciênc. saúde coletiva. n.3 vol.15 Rio de Janeiro May 2010.

SHINKAI, R. S. A.; CURY, A. A. D. B. O papel da odontologia na equipe interdisciplinar: contribuindo para a atenção integral do idoso. Caderno Saúde Pública. Rio de Janeiro, 16(4):1099-1109, October-December, 2000.

TURANO, J. C.; TURANO, M. L. Fundamentals of total prosthesis. 6. ed. São Paulo: Santos, 2002.

XAVIER, A. et al.. Oral condition of an Amazonian population in the interior of the state of Rondônia: use and need for prostheses. Arq. Odontol.; Belo Horizonte, 47 (1): 9-17, Jan/Mar,

2011.

CHAPTER 8
ANNEXES

ANNEX 1 : CEP'S SUBSTANTIATED OPINION

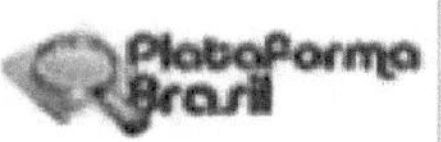

UNIVERSIDADE PAULISTA - UNIP - VICE-REITORIA DE PESQUISA E PÓS

PARECER CONSUBSTANCIADO DO CEP

DADOS DO PROJETO DE PESQUISA

Título da Pesquisa: AVALIAÇÃO DO GRAU DE SATISFAÇÃO DE PACIENTES ATENDIDOS NA CLÍNICA DE PRÓTES TOTAL DA FACULDADE DE ODONTOLOGIA DA UNIP-MANAUS

Pesquisador: NELY CRISTINA MEDEIROS CAIRES
Área Temática:
Versão: 1
CAAE: 06165612.7.0000.5512
Instituição Proponente: Universidade Paulista - UNIP / Vice-Reitoria de Pesquisa e Pós Graduação

DADOS DO PARECER

Número do Parecer: 142.042
Data da Relatoria: 18/10/2012

Apresentação do Projeto:
De acordo

Objetivo da Pesquisa:
De acordo

Avaliação dos Riscos e Benefícios:
Não há riscos

Comentários e Considerações sobre a Pesquisa:
O trabalho interessa na area de odontologia social

Considerações sobre os Termos de apresentação obrigatória:
De acordo

Recomendações:
Nada a acrescentar

Conclusões ou Pendências e Lista de Inadequações:
Não foram observadas inadequações

Situação do Parecer:
Aprovado

INFORMED CONSENT FORM

Dear Participant:

We would like to invite you to participate as a volunteer in the research entitled EVALUATION OF THE DEGREE OF SATISFACTION OF PATIENTS ATTENDED AT THE TOTAL PROSTHESIS CLINIC OF THE FACULTY OF ODONTOLOGY OF UNIP- MANAUS which refers to a Scientific Initiation project of the participant(s) JOSEANE FROTA MENDES DE ARAUJO of the Graduation, which belongs to the Course of ODONTOLOGY of the UNIVERSIDADE PAULISTA CAMPUS MANAUS.

The aim(s) of this study is to assess the level of satisfaction with the total prosthesis of patients treated at the Teaching Dentistry Clinic of the UNIP Manaus campus. The results will help us to evaluate the positive and negative aspects of the care provided to patients who have had their total prosthesis made at the UNIP-MANAUS Prosthesis Clinic.

Their form of participation consists of taking part in a questionnaire about satisfaction with the total prosthesis and a clinical examination of it.

Your name will not be used at any stage of the research, which guarantees your anonymity, and the results will be publicised in such a way as not to identify the volunteers.

There will be no charge, no expenses and no compensation.

Considering that all research offers some kind of risk, in this research the risk can be assessed as: minimal

The following immediate benefits are expected from your participation in this research: Evaluation of the total prosthesis in use and referral for adjustments if necessary.

We would like to make it clear that your participation is voluntary and that you may refuse to participate or withdraw your consent, or discontinue your participation if you so choose, without any penalty or prejudice to your care.

Thank you in advance for your attention and participation, and we remain at your disposal for further information.

You will keep a copy of this Agreement and if you have any questions or clarifications about this research you can contact the principal investigator, NELY CRISTINA MEDEIROS CAIRES, TEL: 92 8187 0595.

I (participant's name and identity document number) confirm that NELT CRISTINA MEDEIROS CAIRES, JOSEANE FROTA MENDES DE ARAUJO have explained the objectives of this research to me, as well as how to participate. The alternatives to my participation were also discussed. I have read and understood this consent form, so I agree to give my consent to participate as a volunteer in this research.

Place and date: MANAUS, 29th July 2011.

____

(Signature of research subject or legal representative)

____

(Signature of witness for illiterate, semi-literate or hearing, visual or motor impaired subjects).

Me, ____

(name of the team member presenting the ICF)

I properly and voluntarily obtained the Free and Informed Consent of the research subject or legal representative to participate in the research.

____

(Signature of the team member presenting the ICF)

____

(Identification and signature of the researcher in charge)

ANNEX 3: Patient Identification.

Age:

65 to 70 ( ) 71 to 75 ( ) 76 to 80 ( ) 80 or more ( )

Gender:

Male (1) Female (2)

Time he lost his teeth ____

Wears full dentures: Yes (1) No (2)

Top ( ) Bottom ( ) The Pair ( )

For how long? ____

ANNEX4: OHIP-14 DIMENSIONS FOR PORTUGUESE LANGUAGE

	In the last six months	Never (D	Almost never (2)	Sometimes (3)	Fairly often (4)	Often (5)
Limitation Functional	1.Have you had problems speaking a word because of problems with your teeth, mouth or dentures?					
	2. Have you experienced a change in taste due to problems with your teeth, mouth or dentures?					
Pain	3. Have you experienced severe pain in your mouth?					
Physics	4. Have you felt uncomfortable					

	eating food because of problems with your teeth, mouth or dentures?					
Discomfort Psychological	5. Are you worried about problems with your teeth, mouth or dentures?					
	6. Have you felt stressed because of problems with your teeth, mouth or dentures?					
Inability Physics	7.Has eating been impaired because of problems with your teeth, mouth or dentures?					
	8.Have you had to stop eating because of problems with your teeth, mouth or dentures?					
Inability Psychological	9.Have you found it difficult to relax because of problems with your teeth, mouth or dentures?					
	10. Have you felt embarrassed because of problems with your teeth, mouth or dentures?					
Inability Social	11. Have you been irritated by other people because of problems with your teeth, mouth or dentures?					
	12. Difficulties carrying out your daily activities because of problems with your teeth, mouth or dentures?					
Physical Limitation	13 Have you felt that life in general has become worse because of problems with your teeth, mouth or dentures?					
	14.Have you been totally unable to carry out your daily activities because of problems with your teeth, mouth or dentures?					

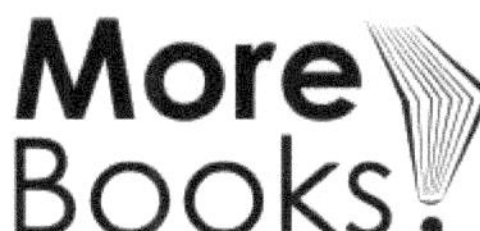

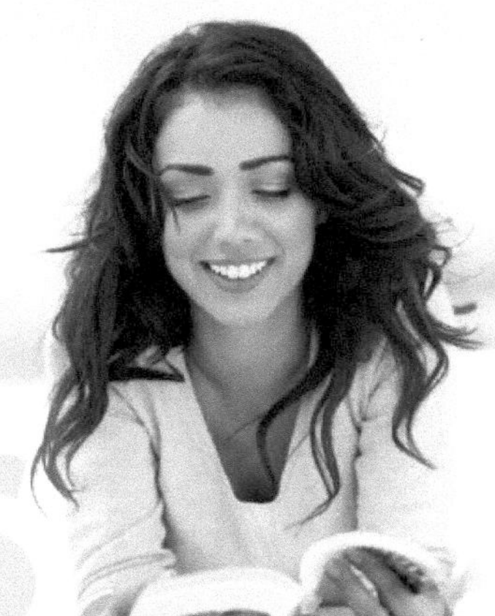

I want morebooks!

Buy your books fast and straightforward online - at one of world's fastest growing online book stores! Environmentally sound due to Print-on-Demand technologies.

Buy your books online at
www.morebooks.shop

Kaufen Sie Ihre Bücher schnell und unkompliziert online – auf einer der am schnellsten wachsenden Buchhandelsplattformen weltweit! Dank Print-On-Demand umwelt- und ressourcenschonend produziert.

Bücher schneller online kaufen
www.morebooks.shop

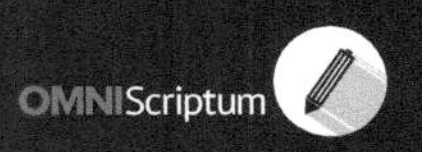

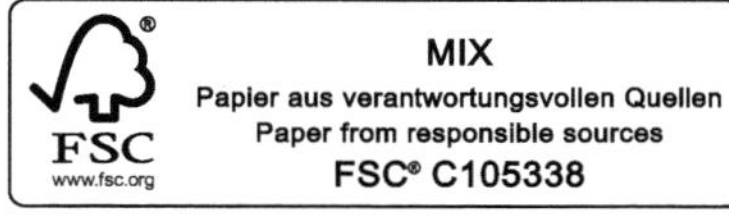

Printed by Books on Demand GmbH, Norderstedt / Germany